THE HIATAL HERNIA COOKING GUIDE FOR SENIORS.

Defeating hiatal hernia with food with age factors in consideration.

Michelle Apron

Table of contents

INTRODUCTION

A hiatal hernia is a common condition that occurs when part of the stomach bulges up through an opening in the diaphragm, the muscle that separates the abdomen from the chest. This opening, called the esophageal hiatus, is normally small enough to allow only the esophagus to pass through. However, in people with a hiatal hernia, the opening is larger, allowing part of the stomach to slip up into the chest cavity.

The diaphragm is a huge muscle that is located between your abdomen and chest. You use this muscle to help you breathe. Normally, your stomach is below the diaphragm, but in people with a hiatal hernia, a portion of the stomach pushes up through the muscle. The opening it moves through is known as a hiatus.

Types of Hiatal Hernia

Sliding hiatal hernia

About 95% of occurrences of hiatal hernias are of the sliding variety, which is the most prevalent kind. The esophagogastric junction (EGJ), which connects the esophagus and stomach, slips up into the chest through the diaphragm's hole in a sliding hiatal hernia. Heartburn, regurgitation, and other symptoms of acid reflux disease (GERD) may result from this.

Paraesophageal hiatal hernia

Approximately 5% of occurrences of hiatal hernias are of this less prevalent variety. A portion of the stomach rises up through the diaphragm's hole next to the esophagus in a paraesophageal hiatal hernia. Complications from this kind of hernia are more likely to occur, including bleeding or incarceration (when the hernia gets lodged in the chest).

CHAPTER ONE

Hiatal Hernia and seniors

Although hiatal hernias can happen to anyone at any age, they are far more common as people age, especially in those over 60. The significant influence of age-related changes on the diaphragm and its supporting components is highlighted by this increased occurrence.

Factors Associated with Age that Cause Hiatal Hernia

There are various age-related factors that contribute to the higher incidence of hiatal hernia in older persons, including:

Diaphragmatic Weakening: The muscles and connective tissues of the diaphragm gradually lose their flexibility and resilience as we age. The stomach might protrude through the gap as a result of the diaphragm becoming weaker and more prone to herniation.

Alterations in Connective Tissue: As we age, our connective tissue—the structural foundation that supports our tissues and organs—becomes less resilient and more prone to stretching. Hiatal hernia development is facilitated by this weakness.

Increased Abdominal Pressure: As people age, they are more likely to experience the effects of obesity, persistent coughing, and hard lifting, among other factors that tend to raise abdominal pressure. The weaker diaphragm is subjected to additional strain by this elevated pressure, increasing the risk of herniation.

Symptoms in Elderly Adults and How to Manage Them

Depending on the extent of diaphragmatic weakness and the size of the hernia, hiatal hernias may or may not cause symptoms. When symptoms do appear, though, they are usually linked to acid reflux, a disorder in which stomach acid refluxes back into the esophagus. The following are typical signs of a hiatal hernia:

Heartburn: The most common sign of acid reflux is a burning feeling in the chest, which is brought on by stomach acid's irritating effects on the lining of the esophagus.

Regurgitation: One of the most common signs of a hiatal hernia is the involuntary flow of stomach contents—such as acid, food, or liquid—back up into the mouth.

Dysphagia, or difficulty swallowing, is a common condition in older persons. It is caused by a weaker diaphragm and changes to the structure of the esophagus.

Chest discomfort: If chest discomfort is accompanied by regurgitation or heartburn, it may indicate a hiatal hernia.

A test or treatment to identify the reason of upper abdomen or chest pain, or heartburn, frequently reveals a hiatal hernia. These examinations or methods consist of:

an upper gastrointestinal X-ray. After consuming a gritty liquid that coats and fills the interior lining of your digestive tract, X-rays are taken. Your doctor can see a silhouette of your stomach, upper intestines, and esophagus thanks to the coating.

upper endoscopy. Your doctor will place an endoscope—a small, flexible tube with a light and camera—down your throat to see inside your stomach and esophagus and assess for inflammation.

gastroscopy manometry. The test gauges the regular contractions of the muscles in your esophagus during swallowing. Esophageal manometry additionally assesses the force and synchronization of your esophageal muscles.

CHAPTER TWO

HOW DIET COMES TO THE RESCUE

Stomach acids can more easily pass through the esophagus, which is the tube that transports food from your throat to your stomach, if you have a hiatal hernia. Your chest and throat start to burn as a result. For certain people, certain foods can exacerbate these symptoms. Fortunately, dietary and lifestyle modifications can frequently alleviate the heartburn symptoms linked to hiatal hernias.

Nutritional Guidelines for Hiatal Hernias

Eat Less Acidic meals: Acidic meals can exacerbate the symptoms of a hiatal hernia and cause heartburn. Citrus fruits, tomatoes, tomato-based sauces, vinegar, and fizzy drinks are among them.

Limit Fatty and Spicy Foods: These foods can exacerbate heartburn symptoms by slowing down digestion and producing more stomach acid.

Steer clear of alcohol and caffeine: These substances have the ability to relax the lower esophageal sphincter (LES), which is the valve that separates the stomach from the esophagus. This increases the likelihood that stomach acid will reflux.

Eat Smaller, Frequent Meals: Consuming large meals might exacerbate reflux by applying additional pressure to the LES. Choose to eat smaller, more frequent meals throughout the day as an alternative.

Eat Slowly and Chew Carefully: Proper digestion facilitates a lighter stomach and less strain on the LES when food is consumed slowly and completely chewed.

Keep Your Weight in Check: Being overweight can increase the pressure on the abdomen and exacerbate the symptoms of a hiatal hernia. Try to maintain a healthy weight to ease this strain.

Raise the Head of Your Bed: When you're lying down, it's easier for stomach acid to reflux back into your esophagus. This can be avoided by raising the head of your bed by 6 to 8 inches.

Refrain from Lying Down Immediately After Meals: To lower the chance of acid reflux, wait at least three hours after eating before lying down.

Put on loose-fitting attire: Wearing clothing that is too tight might compress the abdomen and exacerbate the symptoms of a hiatal hernia. Choose clothing that fits loosely around the waist.

Reduce Stress: Stress can make the symptoms of a hiatal hernia worse. Look for stress-reduction techniques that are beneficial, like yoga, meditation, or exercise.

Cooking the meals that will be included in this book in a healthful manner is a great way to enjoy them. Here are some culinary advice that could help prevent heartburn:

Pick lean meats like fish, skinless chicken, meat with minimal visible fat, and ground turkey rather than ground beef. Chuck, loin, sirloin, and round are examples of lean beef cuts. Tenderloin and loin chop are examples of lean pig cuts.

Foods can be baked or broiler instead of fried.

Remove excess fat from meat while it's cooking.

Don't add too much seasoning. As long as they're not hot, most seasonings are safe to use, but only in little amounts.

Instead of ice cream, try low-fat dairy products like low-fat yogurt.

Steam your veggies using just water.

Cut back on oils, butter, and cream sauces. When sautéing, use cooking spray rather than cooking oil.

Select ingredients that are low or nonfat instead of full-fat items.

Use your imagination. There are countless methods for adjusting recipes. Never be scared to attempt new things.

CHAPTER THREE

Here, your easy breakfast recipes

Living with a hiatal hernia can make choosing breakfast options tricky. But worry not, delicious and gentle-on-the-stomach meals are still within reach! Here are 20 breakfast recipes with instructions, tailored for hiatal hernia patients:

1. Oatmeal with Berries and Nuts:

Ingredients:

- 1/2 cup rolled oats
- 1 cup milk or water
- 1/4 cup mixed berries (fresh or frozen)
- 1/4 cup chopped nuts (such as almonds, walnuts, or pecans)

- Honey or maple syrup to taste (optional)

Instructions:

1. In a saucepan, combine oats and milk or water. Bring to a boil, then reduce heat and simmer for 5 minutes, stirring occasionally.
2. Stir in berries and nuts.
3. Serve warm, topped with honey or maple syrup if desired.

2. Scrambled Eggs with Spinach:

Ingredients:

- 2 eggs
- 1 tablespoon milk or water
- 1/4 cup chopped fresh spinach
- Salt and pepper to taste

Instructions:

1. In a bowl, whisk together eggs and milk or water.
2. Heat a small skillet over medium heat. Add spinach and cook until wilted, about 1 minute.
3. Pour egg mixture into the skillet and cook, stirring occasionally, until eggs are set, about 3 minutes.
4. Season with salt and pepper to taste.

3. Greek Yogurt with Honey and Fruit:

Ingredients:

- 1 cup Greek yogurt
- 1 tablespoon honey
- 1/2 cup mixed berries (fresh or frozen)
- 1/4 cup granola (optional)

Instructions:

1. In a bowl, combine yogurt and honey.
2. Top with berries and granola, if desired.

4. Chia Seed Pudding:

Ingredients:

- 1/4 cup chia seeds
- 1 cup milk or almond milk
- 1 tablespoon honey
- 1/2 teaspoon vanilla extract
- 1/4 cup mixed berries (fresh or frozen)

Instructions:

1. In a jar or bowl, combine chia seeds, milk, honey, and vanilla extract. Stir well.
2. Refrigerate overnight, or for at least 2 hours.
3. Stir in berries before serving.

5. Baked Sweet Potato Toast with Avocado:

Ingredients:

- 1 medium sweet potato
- 1/4 avocado, mashed
- Salt and pepper to taste

Instructions:

1. Preheat oven to 400 degrees F (200 degrees C).

2. Pierce sweet potato with a fork and bake for 45-60 minutes, or until tender.
3. Let cool slightly, then slice in half lengthwise.
4. Spread mashed avocado on each half of the sweet potato.
5. Season with salt and pepper to taste.

6. Banana Pancakes:

Ingredients:

- 1 ripe banana, mashed
- 2 eggs
- 1/4 teaspoon baking powder
- Cinnamon or nutmeg to taste (optional)

Instructions:

1. In a bowl, mash the banana.

2. Whisk in the eggs, baking powder, and cinnamon or nutmeg (if using).
3. Heat a lightly greased griddle or skillet over medium heat.
4. Pour batter onto the griddle, forming pancakes of your desired size.
5. Cook for 2-3 minutes per side, or until golden brown.

7. Smoothie with Spinach, Banana, and Berries:

Ingredients:

- 1 cup spinach
- 1 banana, frozen or fresh
- 1/2 cup mixed berries (frozen or fresh)
- 1 cup milk or yogurt

Instructions:

1. Combine all ingredients in a
   blender and blend until smooth.

8. Poached Eggs on Whole-Wheat Toast:

Ingredients:

- 2 eggs
- 1 tablespoon vinegar
- 2 slices whole-wheat toast
- Butter or avocado (optional)

Instructions:

1. Fill a saucepan with water and
   bring to a simmer. Add vinegar.
2. Crack each egg into a small bowl.
   Swirl the water gently to create a
   vortex.
3. Carefully slide each egg into the
   simmering water. Cook for 3-4

minutes, or until whites are set
and yolks are desired doneness.
4. Drain eggs on paper towels.
5. Toast the bread and spread with
butter or avocado, if desired.
6. Top with poached eggs and enjoy.

**9. Cottage Cheese with Fruit and
Honey:**

Ingredients:

- 1/2 cup cottage cheese
- 1/4 cup chopped fruit (such as
mango, pineapple, or
strawberries)
- 1 tablespoon honey

Instructions:

1. In a bowl, combine cottage
cheese and fruit.

2. Drizzle with honey and mix well.

10. Rice Cakes with Almond Butter and Sliced Banana:

Ingredients:

- 2 rice cakes
- 2 tablespoons almond butter
- 1/2 banana, sliced

Instructions:

1. Spread almond butter on each rice cake.
2. Top with sliced banana.

CHAPTER FOUR

Here, your lunch recipes

Day 1: Creamy Roasted Butternut Squash Soup with Toasted Walnuts

Ingredients:

- 1 medium butternut squash, peeled and cubed
- 1 tablespoon olive oil
- 1/2 teaspoon dried thyme
- Salt and pepper to taste
- 1 cup vegetable broth
- 1/2 cup coconut milk (unsweetened)
- 1/4 cup chopped walnuts, toasted

Instructions:

1. Preheat oven to 400°F (200°C). Toss butternut squash with olive oil, thyme, salt, and pepper.

Spread on a baking sheet and roast for 25-30 minutes, or until tender.

2. In a blender, combine roasted squash, vegetable broth, and coconut milk. Blend until smooth and creamy.

3. Heat soup in a pot over medium heat. Adjust seasoning if needed. Top with toasted walnuts before serving.

Day 2: Tuna Salad on Avocado Toast with Lemon Dill Dressing

Ingredients:

- 2 slices whole-wheat bread
- 1 avocado, thinly sliced
- 1 can tuna packed in water, drained and flaked
- 1/4 cup plain Greek yogurt
- 1 tablespoon chopped fresh dill
- 1 tablespoon lemon juice
- Salt and pepper to taste

Instructions:

1. Toast bread and top with avocado slices.
2. In a bowl, combine tuna, Greek yogurt, dill, lemon juice, salt, and pepper. Mix well.
3. Spread tuna salad on top of avocado toast and enjoy.

Day 3: Chicken and Quinoa Stuffed Peppers

Ingredients:

- 2 bell peppers, halved and seeded
- 1 cup cooked quinoa
- 1 (4 oz) boneless, skinless chicken breast, cooked and shredded
- 1/2 cup chopped onion
- 1/2 cup chopped tomato
- 1/4 cup chopped fresh parsley
- 1/4 cup low-fat mozzarella cheese, shredded
- Salt and pepper to taste

Instructions:

1. Preheat oven to 375°F (190°C). Cook quinoa according to package instructions.
2. Saute onion and tomato in a pan with a little olive oil until softened. Stir in cooked chicken, quinoa, parsley, salt, and pepper.
3. Fill bell pepper halves with chicken mixture and top with mozzarella cheese.
4. Bake for 20-25 minutes, or until cheese is melted and bubbly.

Day 4: Salmon with Roasted Asparagus and Brown Rice

Ingredients:

- 1 salmon fillet (4 oz)
- 1 tablespoon olive oil
- Salt and pepper to taste
- 1 bunch asparagus, trimmed
- 1 cup cooked brown rice

- 1/4 cup chopped fresh dill (optional)

Instructions:

1. Preheat oven to 400°F (200°C). Season salmon with olive oil, salt, and pepper.
2. Toss asparagus with olive oil, salt, and pepper. Spread on a baking sheet and roast for 10-15 minutes.
3. While asparagus roasts, pan-sear salmon fillet until cooked through (about 5-7 minutes per side).
4. Plate salmon with roasted asparagus and brown rice. Garnish with dill if desired.

Day 5: Lentil Soup with Whole Wheat Croutons

Ingredients:

- 1 cup brown lentils, rinsed
- 4 cups vegetable broth

- 1/2 cup chopped onion
- 1/2 cup chopped carrots
- 1/2 cup chopped celery
- 2 cloves garlic, minced
- 2 tablespoons olive oil
- 1 teaspoon dried thyme
- Salt and pepper to taste
- 2 slices whole-wheat bread, cubed and toasted

Instructions:

1. In a pot, combine lentils, broth, onion, carrots, celery, garlic, olive oil, and thyme. Bring to a boil, then reduce heat and simmer for 20-25 minutes, or until lentils are tender.
2. Season with salt and pepper to taste.
3. Serve soup with toasted whole wheat croutons.

Day 6: Turkey and Vegetable Lettuce Wraps:

- Ingredients: 4 large lettuce leaves, 1/2 cup cooked ground turkey, 1/4 cup chopped bell pepper, 1/4 cup chopped cucumber, 1/4 cup chopped carrot, 2 tablespoons hummus, 1 tablespoon chopped fresh cilantro.
- Instructions: Wash and dry lettuce leaves. In a bowl, combine ground turkey, bell pepper, cucumber, carrot, hummus, and cilantro. Divide mixture evenly between lettuce leaves and enjoy.

Day 7: Baked Potato with Black Bean Salsa:

- Ingredients: 1 medium potato, 1/2 cup canned black beans, rinsed and drained, 1/4 cup chopped tomato, 1/4 cup chopped red onion, 1 tablespoon chopped fresh cilantro, 1/2 lime, juiced, 1/4 teaspoon chili powder, pinch of salt and pepper.

- Instructions: Preheat oven to 400°F (200°C). Bake potato for 45-50 minutes, or until tender. While potato bakes, combine black beans, tomato, onion, cilantro, lime juice, chili powder, salt, and pepper in a bowl. Slice open baked potato and top with black bean salsa.

Day 8: Creamy Miso Noodle Soup with Tofu:

- Ingredients: 1 cup vegetable broth, 1 tablespoon miso paste, 1/2 cup cooked udon noodles, 1/2 block firm tofu, cubed, 1/4 cup sliced mushrooms, 1/4 cup chopped green onions, 1 tablespoon chopped fresh ginger.
- Instructions: Bring broth to a simmer in a pot. Whisk in miso paste until dissolved. Add

noodles, tofu, mushrooms, green onions, and ginger. Simmer for 5-7 minutes, or until heated through.

Day 9: Chicken and Veggie Quinoa Bowl:

- Ingredients: 1 cup cooked quinoa, 1 (4 oz) boneless, skinless chicken breast, cooked and shredded, 1/2 cup roasted vegetables (e.g., carrots, broccoli, cauliflower), 1/4 cup chopped cucumber, 1/4 cup chopped tomato, 1 tablespoon olive oil, 1 tablespoon lemon juice, salt and pepper to taste.
- Instructions: Combine quinoa, chicken, roasted vegetables, cucumber, and tomato in a bowl. Drizzle with olive oil and lemon juice. Season with salt and pepper to taste.

Day 10: Greek Yogurt Parfait with Fruit and Granola:

- Ingredients: 1 cup plain Greek yogurt, 1/2 cup chopped fruit (e.g., berries, melon, apple), 1/4 cup granola, 1 tablespoon honey (optional).
- Instructions: Layer Greek yogurt, fruit, and granola in a parfait glass. Drizzle with honey if desired.

CHAPTER FIVE

Dinner recipes

1. Salmon with Roasted Vegetables and Quinoa:

Ingredients:

- 1 salmon fillet (6 oz)
- 1 tablespoon olive oil
- 1/2 teaspoon dried thyme
- Salt and pepper to taste
- 1 cup Brussels sprouts, halved
- 1/2 cup red onion, chopped
- 1/2 cup quinoa, rinsed

Instructions:

1. Preheat oven to 400°F (200°C).
2. Season salmon with olive oil, thyme, salt, and pepper.

3. Toss Brussels sprouts and onion
   with olive oil, salt, and pepper.
   Spread on a baking sheet and
   roast for 15 minutes.
4. Add salmon to the baking sheet
   and roast for another 10-15
   minutes, or until salmon is cooked
   through.
5. Meanwhile, cook quinoa
   according to package
   instructions.
6. Serve salmon with roasted
   vegetables and quinoa.

2. Turkey Meatloaf with Sweet Potato Mash:

Ingredients:

- 1 lb ground turkey
- 1/2 cup breadcrumbs
- 1/4 cup milk
- 1 egg, beaten
- 1/2 onion, chopped
- 1 clove garlic, minced

- 1/2 teaspoon dried sage
- Salt and pepper to taste
- 2 sweet potatoes, peeled and chopped
- 1/4 cup milk
- 1 tablespoon butter
- Salt and pepper to taste

Instructions:

1. Preheat oven to 375°F (190°C).
2. Combine ground turkey, breadcrumbs, milk, egg, onion, garlic, sage, salt, and pepper in a bowl. Mix well and form into a loaf.
3. Place meatloaf on a baking sheet and bake for 45 minutes.
4. While meatloaf is cooking, boil sweet potatoes until tender. Drain and mash with milk and butter. Season with salt and pepper.
5. Serve meatloaf with sweet potato mash.

3. Chicken Stir-Fry with Brown Rice:

Ingredients:

- 1 lb boneless, skinless chicken breast, thinly sliced
- 1 tablespoon vegetable oil
- 1 tablespoon soy sauce
- 1 tablespoon honey
- 1 teaspoon ginger, minced
- 1/2 teaspoon garlic powder
- 1 bell pepper, sliced
- 1 broccoli florets
- 1 cup brown rice, cooked

Instructions:

1. In a bowl, combine chicken, soy sauce, honey, ginger, and garlic powder. Marinate for at least 30 minutes.
2. Heat oil in a wok or large skillet over medium heat. Add chicken and cook until browned on all sides.

3. Add bell pepper and broccoli and cook until crisp-tender.
4. Serve stir-fry over brown rice.

4. Baked Cod with Lemon and Herbs:

Ingredients:

- 4 cod fillets (6 oz each)
- 1 tablespoon olive oil
- 1 lemon, sliced
- 1/4 cup fresh herbs (dill, parsley, thyme)
- Salt and pepper to taste

Instructions:

1. Preheat oven to 400°F (200°C).
2. Arrange cod fillets in a baking dish. Drizzle with olive oil and season with salt and pepper.
3. Top each fillet with lemon slices and sprinkle with herbs.
4. Bake for 15-20 minutes, or until cod is cooked through.

5. Lentil Soup with Whole Wheat Bread:

Ingredients:

- 1 tablespoon olive oil
- 1 onion, chopped
- 1 carrot, chopped
- 2 celery stalks, chopped
- 2 cloves garlic, minced
- 1 cup green lentils, rinsed
- 4 cups vegetable broth
- 1 (14.5 oz) can diced tomatoes, undrained
- 1 teaspoon dried oregano
- Salt and pepper to taste
- Whole wheat bread for dipping

Instructions:

1. Heat olive oil in a large pot over medium heat. Add onion, carrot, and celery and cook until softened, about 5 minutes.

2. Add garlic and cook for 1 minute more.
3. Add lentils, broth, tomatoes, and oregano. Bring to a boil, then reduce heat and simmer for 30 minutes, or until lentils are tender.
4. Season with salt and pepper to taste.
5. Serve soup with whole wheat bread for dipping.

6. Creamy Chicken and Rice Casserole:

Ingredients:

- 1 lb boneless, skinless chicken breast, cooked and chopped
- 1 cup cooked brown rice
- 1/2 cup low-fat sour cream
- 1/4 cup milk
- 1/4 cup grated Parmesan cheese
- 1 tablespoon olive oil
- 1 onion, chopped
- 1/2 teaspoon dried thyme

- Salt and pepper to taste

Instructions:

1. Preheat oven to 375°F (190°C).
2. Heat olive oil in a skillet over medium heat. Add onion and cook until softened, about 5 minutes.
3. Add thyme and cook for 1 minute more.
4. In a bowl, combine chicken, rice, sour cream, milk, Parmesan cheese, onion mixture, salt, and pepper.
5. Transfer mixture to a baking dish and bake for 20-25 minutes, or until bubbly and heated through.

7. Shrimp Scampi with Zucchini Noodles:

Ingredients:

- 1 lb large shrimp, peeled and deveined

- 1 tablespoon olive oil
- 2 cloves garlic, minced
- 1/4 cup white wine (optional)
- 1/2 cup chicken broth
- 1/4 cup lemon juice
- 1/4 teaspoon dried oregano
- Salt and pepper to taste
- 2 zucchini, spiralized into noodles

Instructions:

1. Heat olive oil in a large skillet over medium heat. Add garlic and cook for 30 seconds.
2. Add shrimp and cook until pink and cooked through, about 3-4 minutes per side.
3. Remove shrimp from the skillet and set aside.
4. Add white wine (if using) and chicken broth to the skillet. Bring to a simmer and cook until reduced by half, about 5 minutes.
5. Add lemon juice, oregano, salt, and pepper.

6. Add zucchini noodles and cook for 1-2 minutes, until warm and slightly softened.
7. Add shrimp back to the skillet and toss to combine.
8. Serve immediately.

8. Baked Tofu with Roasted Brussels Sprouts:

Ingredients:

- 1 block firm tofu, drained and pressed
- 1 tablespoon olive oil
- 1 tablespoon soy sauce
- 1 teaspoon sriracha (optional)
- 1/2 teaspoon dried rosemary
- Salt and pepper to taste
- 1 pound Brussels sprouts, trimmed and halved
- 1 tablespoon olive oil
- Salt and pepper to taste

Instructions:

1. Preheat oven to 400°F (200°C).
2. Cut tofu into cubes.
3. In a bowl, combine olive oil, soy sauce, sriracha (if using), rosemary, salt, and pepper. Toss tofu cubes in the mixture to coat.
4. Spread tofu cubes on a baking sheet and bake for 20-25 minutes, or until golden brown and crispy.
5. Meanwhile, toss Brussels sprouts with olive oil, salt, and pepper. Spread on a separate baking sheet and roast for 15-20 minutes, or until tender and browned.
6. Serve tofu cubes with roasted Brussels sprouts.

9. Turkey Stuffed Sweet Potatoes:

Ingredients:

- 2 large sweet potatoes
- 1 pound ground turkey
- 1/2 cup diced onion
- 1/2 cup chopped celery

- 1/2 cup chopped bell pepper
- 1 clove garlic, minced
- 1/2 cup cooked quinoa
- 1/4 cup low-fat yogurt
- 1/4 cup chopped fresh parsley
- 1/2 teaspoon dried sage
- Salt and pepper to taste

Instructions:

1. Preheat oven to 400°F (200°C).
2. Pierce sweet potatoes with a fork and microwave for 5 minutes to soften slightly. Cut in half and scoop out the flesh, leaving a 1/2-inch border.
3. Heat olive oil in a skillet over medium heat. Add onion, celery, and bell pepper and cook until softened, about 5 minutes.
4. Add ground turkey and cook until browned. Add garlic and cook for 1 minute more.
5. In a bowl, combine cooked sweet potato flesh, quinoa, yogurt,

parsley, sage, salt, and pepper. Mix in with the ground turkey mixture.

6. Fill sweet potato shells with the stuffing and bake for 20-25 minutes, or until heated through.

TIPS AND DAILY LIFESTYLE

Although there isn't a treatment for hiatal hernias, there are several ways to manage your symptoms and stop them from growing worse.

Modifications in lifestyle

Consume smaller meals more often. By doing this, you can lessen the strain on your stomach and keep it from pressing into your diaphragm.

Steer clear of fat and spicy food. These meals may worsen your symptoms by irritating the lining of your stomach.

Avoid eating or drinking right before bed. This can help prevent heartburn by giving your stomach time to empty before you lie down.

Raise the head of your mattress. By doing this, you can lessen the chance of stomach contents spilling into your esophagus.

Put on loose-fitting attire. Wearing tight clothing can exacerbate your discomfort by applying more pressure to your stomach.

If you are obese or overweight, lose weight. Reducing your weight, even a little bit, can ease the pressure on your stomach.

Give up smoking. Smoking may aggravate the lining of your stomach and exacerbate your symptoms.

Control your tension. Stress can exacerbate symptoms of hiatal hernias. Look for healthy stress-reduction techniques, including yoga, meditation, or physical activity.

Medications available without a prescription

Heartburn relief and stomach acid neutralization are two benefits of antacid use.

H2 blockers have the potential to lessen stomach acid production.

Heartburn medications that are the most effective are proton pump inhibitors.

prescription drugs

Should over-the-counter treatments prove insufficient in managing your symptoms, your physician may recommend a more potent medication.

Operation

Surgery is often only contemplated in cases where medicines and lifestyle modifications are ineffective in managing your symptoms. Restoring the hiatal hernia and stopping the stomach from pushing through the diaphragm are the two main objectives of surgery.

Extra advice

Give your food a good chew. This will facilitate the easier digestion of your food in your stomach by breaking it down.

Steer clear of carbonated drinks. These drinks may aggravate your symptoms by causing gas and bloating.

Make sure to stay hydrated. Drinking fluids can help prevent constipation, which can place additional strain on your stomach, and keep your stools smooth.

Elevate your bed's head. By doing this, you can lessen the chance of stomach contents spilling into your esophagus.

Put on loose-fitting attire. Wearing tight clothing can exacerbate your discomfort by applying more pressure to your stomach.

MEAL PLANNER

	BREAKFAST	LUNCH	DINNER
MON			
TUE			
WED			

THU

FRI

SAT

SUN			

	BREAKFAST	LUNCH	DINNER
MON			
TUE			

WED			
THU			
FRI			

SAT			

SUN			

	BREAKFAST	LUNCH	DINNER
MON			

TUE			
WED			
THU			

FRI			
SAT			
SUN			

	BREAKFAST	LUNCH	DINNER

MON			
TUE			
WED			

THU			
FRI			
SAT			

SUN			

	BREAKFAST	LUNCH	DINNER
MON			
TUE			

WED			
THU			
FRI			

SAT			
SUN			

	BREAKFAST	LUNCH	DINNER
MON			

TUE			
WED			
THU			

FRI			
SAT			
SUN			

	BREAKFAST	LUNCH	DINNER

MON			
TUE			
WED			

THU			
FRI			
SAT			

SUN			

	BREAKFAST	LUNCH	DINNER
MON			
TUE			

WED			
THU			
FRI			

	BREAKFAST	LUNCH	DINNER
SAT			
SUN			

	BREAKFAST	LUNCH	DINNER
MON			

TUE			
WED			
THU			

FRI			
SAT			
SUN			

www.ingramcontent.com/pod-product-compliance
Lightning Source LLC
Chambersburg PA
CBHW061014260726

48661CB00005B/2185